SHED THE MINDSET SHED THE POUNDS

8 Easy Steps That Will Promote Weight Loss

COURTNEY F. MOORE

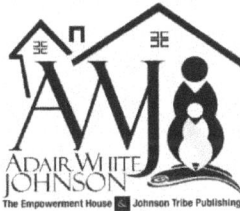

ADAIR WHITE JOHNSON
The Empowerment House | Johnson Tribe Publishing

Acknowledgments

Life has offered many challenges to date, which I viewed as opportunities, not because I'm so inclined but, because my parents have instilled this perspective.

I would like to give thanks to my parents,

Aston and Ouida (Dotty) Moore

Contents

Foreword

From a size 32 waist to a size 44 waist right In front of my eyes, being diagnosed with obesity, hypertension, diabetes, and other medical conditions, was an astounding reality, for this former athlete.... the author. I have known the author for many years and witnessed his rapid weight gain and unhealthy lifestyle choices, which precipitated the authors need for medical intervention. Based on my experience, I was also well aware that Courtney's medical issues were unfortunately not uncommon, however. As a healthcare professional, I am aware that a high incidence of obesity, hypertension, diabetes, etc., does exist, and how it can and does impact the individual as well as the family.

Shed the mindset shed the pounds, will give you, the reader, a raw, unapologetic level of brutal honesty of the author's medical crisis, his personal perspectives on healthcare, the food industry and how he fought like hell for his life. The book is a cathartic unveiling of the author's pain, fears and the fight or flight instinct that propelled Courtney to lose 65 pounds in 6 months. Read on about the 8 steps the author took to achieve his personal weight loss goal. More importantly, see the lifestyle change the author implemented to successfully and drastically improve his health. With this book, you can be empowered to conquer your weight loss goal, too!

Jacqueline Gibbons, LMSW

Preface

When I think of weight loss, an old British military term comes to mind, "A shot across the bow." It derives from the naval practice of firing a cannon shot across the bows of an opponent's ship to show them that you are prepared to do battle. The more general figurative use of the expression means warning. Pharses.org.uk. This thought is significant for two reasons, one, I was ready to do battle, lose weight and get healthy and two, almost passing out while attending my son's baseball camp was truly a warning; if I didn't make lifestyle changes, I wouldn't be around much longer to support my family.

I majored in business in graduate school, and one of the concepts I learned was called ESI or early simultaneous influence. It's a process used in business which was developed by one of my professors Dr. Frank Hull. Essentially it takes a look at the entire manufacturing process from the cradle to the grave and is designed to cut cost and save time by concurrently involving several stakeholders early in the process. I have successfully applied these principles to several non-manufacturing projects I have engaged in post-graduate school.

ESI can be applied to and works very well with the weight loss process. In other words, if your goal is to lose weight and get healthy, then no one weight loss concept, diet or exercise plan may be adequate. Also, if your weight loss plan is only followed sporadically, then you are doomed to fail. The solution is simple, apply my eight weight loss techniques simultaneously and run them concurrently to lose weight quickly and keep it off.

First, we have to shed our current mindset to shed the pounds. In other words, employ a paradigm shift. Second, you must cleanse your body; this is the initial step in the diet process and needs to happen before beginning the others. Follow up by implementing the next five steps, remember simultaneously for best results. They are as follows: home remedies, food & diet, Stress relief & meditation, fasting, and exercise & fitness program. Then end your weight loss regimen by employing a weight management program to keep the excess pounds off for good.

Introduction

Impact of Weight Gain and Poor Health on My Life

Somewhere along the way between high school graduation and the present time I gained over 85 pounds. In high school, I was a svelte 155lbs, the captain of both the football and track teams. I was in the best shape of my life fit and as healthy as can be.

One day, several years later, I took my son to a baseball camp at a university in North Carolina and my life changed forever, First for the worst and then for the better in a matter of six months.

Indulge me a little while I set the stage: The baseball field was located up a very steep hill from the parking lot. I dropped my son off at the field parked my car and took off on a journey up the hill. Halfway up I was out of breath and felt like I was going to pass out. My chest got tight, my heart was racing, and I was sweating profusely. Thoughts ran through my mind of dying at my son's baseball camp. I thought about not being around to attend their graduation, weddings or seeing my grandchildren take their first step. Luckily, I was not experiencing a heart attack I was just overweight, out of breath and out of shape.

I decided from that day forward that I was going to make changes to my lifestyle and get healthy. After living a sedentary lifestyle eating whatever I want to and drinking sometimes aimlessly, I embarked on a quest to turn my life around. I knew it would not be easy but if I didn't give it "the old college try" I wouldn't be here to support my family or share my story with you.

The plan was simple: visit my primary care physician (which I have neglected to do in years) and check my numbers. If everything checked out, then I would start an exercise program and some form of a healthy diet.

As stated earlier, things got worse before I was able to turn them around. The day came to see the doctor. She conducted every test known to man. And three days later I was instructed to return to the office for a consultation.

I had never been more terrified in my entire life and for a good reason. My results were poor; they showed a multitude of disorders associated with metabolic syndrome. I was obese (Body Mass Index of 35), I was hypertensive, I had type II diabetes, I had high cholesterol, and I weighed a whopping 240lbs. Just wait, there is more! I was instructed to go and see the Ophthalmologist, the Gastroenterologist, and the Podiatrist.

A little bit of quiet before the storm, I did not have colon cancer nor did I have diabetic foot disease such as Peripheral Neuropathy (Diabetic Nerve Pain). Thank God! I did, however, have a cataract in the right eye and a fast progressing matured white cataract in the left eye that quickly rendered me legally blind for a month until corrected by surgery. I was made aware of the fact that I was several years younger than the typical cataract patient. The early onset of the overall eye disease and the severity of the left eye were due to uncontrolled hypertension and uncontrolled diabetes. Also, the Ophthalmologist indicated that I was suffering from Ischemic Eye Syndrome (lack of blood flow to the back of the eyes) WOW! An ultrasound was conducted to check for carotid artery blockage, and that came back normal as well.

There is still more. I'm embarrassed even to share my thoughts on the next subject. I had a feeling of overall poor health. I had low energy, was fatigued, sluggish at times, out of breath with most activities. Can you imagine the star high school running back not wanting or unable to engage in most physical activities? The only push-ups I did were to push-up the fork to my mouth? If nothing else that was going to change. Oh, and by the way, it did!

After the poor diagnoses there came the prescriptions. My doctor offered no advice on weight loss, no information on how to manage any of my ailments. Instead, she merely prescribed three antidiabetic drugs, one that is very safe and been on the market for over 20 years, a non-insulin injection and a third that is the constant subject of lawsuits. She also prescribed an ACE inhibitor for hypertension and a statin for high cholesterol. I went from taking a multivitamin the day before to five prescription drugs in a matter of minutes. Or did I?

Overwhelmed by this disturbing news or should I say downright scared by it, I decided to conduct research of my own on the prevalence of metabolic syndrome, diabetes, hypertension, high cholesterol and obesity in the US. Additionally, I studied the side effect profile of each of the drugs prescribed to me. My findings were alarming.

Disease States

Metabolic Syndrome:

Let's start by defining metabolic syndrome which encompasses just about all of the above disease states. The Mayo Clinic defines metabolic syndrome as "a cluster of conditions-increased blood pressure, high blood sugar, excess body fat around the waist and abnormal cholesterol or triglyceride levels-that occur together, increasing your risk of heart disease, stroke, and diabetes." Data from the National Health and Nutrition Examination Survey (NHANES) 1999-2006 reported a metabolic syndrome prevalence of 34%.

Diabetes:

Diabetes is a disease that affects your body's ability to either adequately use insulin or produce insulin. There are two primary forms of diabetes, Type I and Type II. For our purposes, we are going to focus on Type II diabetes mainly.

According to the National Diabetes Statistics Report of 2014 conducted by the CDC. 29.1 million people or 9.3% of the U.S. population have diabetes. 21.0 million are diagnosed, and 8.1 million are undiagnosed.

There are several co-existing conditions and complications associated with a diagnosis of diabetes. They include heart disease and stroke, blindness, kidney disease, and lower-limb amputations. Have I gotten your attention yet? While there is no accepted cure, diabetes can be treated and managed by medication, exercise, and healthy eating habits. The key is to slow down if not stop the progression of the disease altogether by developing a healthy lifestyle.

Hypertension:

Hypertension occurs when the pressure of the blood pumping through your arteries is higher than it should be. Having high blood pressure puts you at risk for heart disease and stroke, which are the leading causes of death in the U.S. Do we see a pattern yet? The CDC's fact sheet on hypertension June 2016, States that about 75 million American adults have high blood pressure; that is one in every three adults. Only about half the people with high blood pressure have their condition under control. Alarming!

Hyperlipidemia:

Hyperlipidemia is an abnormally high concentration of fats or lipids in the blood. It's the technical word for a disease more commonly known as high cholesterol. 73.5 million adults in the United States have high low-density lipoprotein (LDL) or "bad" cholesterol. People with high total cholesterol have approximately twice the risk of heart disease as people with ideal levels. Nearly 31 million adults have an overall cholesterol level higher than 240 mg/dl. I extracted this data from the CDC's fact sheet on Hyperlipidemia.

Obesity:

Obesity has been defined by the National Institutes of Health (the NIH) as a BMI (Body Mass Index) of 30 and above, In other words, the condition of being grossly fat or overweight. Another aspect of this syndrome is abdominal obesity, which is the extra fat around the mid-section. Typically, a waist size of 35 or higher in women and 40 and higher in men is a good indication of abdominal obesity.

According to the (NIH) "more than two-thirds (68.8percent) of adults are considered to be overweight or obese. More than one-third (35.7 percent) of adults are considered to be obese. More than 1 in 20 (6.3 percent) have extreme obesity. Almost 3 in 4 men (74 percent) are considered to be overweight or obese." Unbelievable!

I think this paints a pretty grim picture of the overall poor health and disease risk factors of adults in the United States. I didn't mean to put you to sleep with these boring statistics, but I felt it necessary to put this in proper perspective and to emphasize the importance of good health.

The Wonderful World of Prescription Drugs

Next, let's explore the impact of prescription drugs on the United States. Believe me, after reading this section you will see why I decided to take only one medication for diabetes and one for hypertension. I did not take any Statins (cholesterol-lowering drugs).

Physicians are required to take the Hippocratic Oath, and one of the promises within that oath is "first do no harm." Medicine today, however, seems to focus on treating disease with the use of pharmaceuticals rather than curing them or finding alternatives to prescribing harmful medications. Just take a look at my doctor, she very casually said to me "take these five drugs and see me in a month." Why did I pay her a co-pay? A 12-year-old could have given me the same advice. I'm not, however, necessarily blaming physicians for how they engage their patients in today's environment of managed care and rising healthcare costs. The waiting rooms are overcrowded, and reimbursement rates are dropping to name a few obstacles they face daily. Still, I can't help but raise an eyebrow or two for the way some practice medicine today. In a lot of cases, I won't say in all cases though; the pharmaceutical industry has a lot to do with it, for example, they create markets for drugs that they have in their pipeline. Take a look at the overactive bladder market or the erectile dysfunction market. Trust me; Pharmaceutical entities created those markets. First came the drug then came the market. And you know what, that's okay, that's the American way. We, however, have choices though, don't we?

The research and development by the Pharma industry have shifted from finding medicines that cure diseases to drugs/medications that treat the symptoms of diseases for a lifetime. That's if the side effects don't kill you before the condition that they are treating does. While drug companies do a tremendous amount of good, they are, however, pressured to be profitable by their shareholders. The outcome of these practices could result in you being on a drug for your lifetime. This may all sound cynical, but it's very true. If we are looking for cures, we will have to turn to academia for them not pharmaceutical companies, or we have to grab the bull by the horns and do it ourselves.

Have you ever wondered why physicians prescribe products the way that they do? Pharmaceutical companies get to medical students very early in their careers; they purchase textbooks and other medically necessary items for these students and interns. Their members sit on the boards of many advocacy groups that were founded to educate consumers on the health risks associated with diseases. They have physicians who are paid handsomely to give product lectures to other doctors in academia and out in the community. The industry is notorious for sponsoring lecture series and for providing continuing education courses and seminars for doctors.

They flood billions of dollars into the advertisements that come right into your living room. Have you ever seen the cholesterol and diabetes commercials with brightly colored scenery with people smiling, singing and dancing? Why is that?

I will tell you why. It is to get your money.

Have you ever wondered why cholesterol numbers, A1C, and the like frequently change or why or how they calculated them in the first place? I suspect highly paid Pharma physicians probably had something to do with it. Hmm!

Last but not least, the "good old" Pharma rep. Just walk into any physician office and sit there for a while and count. I guarantee you will see no less than 25 well dressed, drop dead gorgeous marketers waiting to tell the doctor every positive aspect about their potentially toxic drug. I am not suggesting that these reps are not highly skilled or very intelligent, but it's all about appearance and marketing. I certainly will never begrudge a person for making a living; I too work in the sales and marketing industry.

Follow the Money

I showed you above the millions of Americans with possible life-limiting diseases that typically lead to heart attack, stroke and even death. If you were in the drug business would you research and develop products that would slow disease progression while not providing a cure? Would you? I'm not sure. Some drugs have very unfavorable side effects that will cause severe damage to your vital organs while costing billions of dollars.

According to Statistics.com, "The United States alone holds over 45 percent of the global pharmaceutical market. In 2016 this share was valued around 446 billion US dollars." When we look at diseases such as diabetes alone, the cost is around 322 billion US dollars according to The American Diabetes Association.

Again, nothing wrong with making money and there is nothing wrong with all the good that pharmaceuticals have done to help people around the world, but there are alternatives to taking toxic medications, especially in the metabolic syndrome arena. For example, diet, exercise, and supplements to name a few.

Before we get into the toxicity of the drugs prescribed for the above ailments, let's take a look at the clever schemes that Pharma companies use to keep the funds flowing in and Americans medicated. When a product goes "off patent," typically generic manufactures develop and launch their own FDA approved version of a drug, which leads to lower costs for the consumer. Not so fast, there is something called a product line extension which is a way for companies to extend the period a product is "on patent" by simply changing the dosing or providing a different delivery method for the same drug. Look at the insulin industry, for example; they have come out with minor improvements or molecular changes to their products that keep them patent protected and drive up costs. In many cases, insulin costs have gone up from under $20 a vial to over $250 without necessarily having better efficacy or better patient outcomes.

Adverse Events

Finally, taking prescriptions such as Statins can lead to an increased risk of liver dysfunction, kidney failure, muscle damage, diabetes, cognitive problems, and fatigue. Just Google any of the cholesterol or diabetes drugs previously mentioned, and you will find multiple lawsuits associated with them. They are still on the market with a new one coming out every month. What's alarming to me is upon further research, studies are all over the globe. Some suggest good long-term outcomes (these studies are usually industry-funded) while others were unable to provide supporting data for better patient outcomes as it relates to cardiovascular deaths. In other words, there are mixed reviews as to whether taking these medications will make you live longer or prevent primary heart attack or stroke.

One night I had trouble sleeping, and I turned on the television, immediately a diabetes commercial came on followed by a class action lawsuit commercial. The lawsuit just happened to be for one of the products prescribed by my physician. The lawyer suggested that the product causes ketoacidosis, kidney failure and can even lead to death. Now am I suggesting not taking medication as prescribed by your physician, absolutely not? I am not qualified to make that assertion. What is important here is to evaluate the risks vs. rewards at least when considering these drugs. In my opinion, what doctors are saying is "take these statin drugs that may reduce your cholesterol yet potentially damage your liver and kidneys in the process. Then I will put you on an additional medication and dialysis right before you die". Reduce your mortality risks, take less toxic drugs and or supplements, diet and exercise, save money and live longer. Hmm, what a noble concept! Don't fund your demise, while lining the pockets of others with gold; merely look for safer and more natural alternatives.

The Flavor of your Food

Now that we have touched on some of the adverse effects of prescription drugs let's explore very briefly how the food industry employs some of the same marketing techniques also used in pharmaceuticals ultimately promoting obesity and overall bad health.

I am sure by now you have heard of the 2015 World Health Organization (WHO) report on processed meat. That's hot dogs, sausages, bacon, and most lunch meats. Let me start off by first telling you what the WHO is all about. The WHO began in 1948 and was constructed to provide a healthier future for people across the globe. They made up of more than 7000 people working in offices in more than 150 countries. In October of 2015 The International Agency for Research on Cancer (IARC) which is the cancer agency of the World Health Organization, has classified processed meats as a carcinogen, in other words, something that causes cancer. You know like cigarettes! They also classified red meat as a probable carcinogen.

I know that we have not mentioned cancer before now but, if you consider how these meats are processed, you will quickly discover that consumption could not only lead to cancer but diseases associated with obesity as well. To smoke, preserve or even flavor these meats all kinds of salt, sugar, and chemicals are added to products already high in saturated fats. And that my friend is a recipe for disaster. I see warnings on cigarette boxes, yet I have never seen a health warning on a pack of bacon. I doubt I ever will.

As with the pharmaceutical industry, some of the advocacy groups are sponsored and endorsed by companies in the food business. Groups that are supposed to warn against the health risks associated with processed foods certainly have so-called healthy recipes on their websites containing some of these items. The reason is pretty apparent, fast food companies, junk food companies as well as processed meat companies pump millions of dollars into the coffer of these groups. Without them most if not all of these groups would fold. They then mislead consumers into purchasing products that will eventually lead to lifelong diseases.

Once again, I am not suggesting that you go cold turkey with meats, fast food or junk food. After all, what would summer be like without a couple of cookouts? Consider healthy alternatives to processed foods before consuming.

Plan of Action

Start by looking in the mirror and ask yourself these questions:

1) Was I in shape in high school?
2) How did I look when I met my significant other? Or am I complacent now that I have a significant other?
3) Have I accepted my condition and ailments as a natural part of aging?
4) Have I put work before my health?
5) Have I taken care of everyone in my family, kids, parents and neglected myself?

The answer is probably yes to most if not all of the above questions. Let's do something about it. Now we will discuss my approach to weight loss and the methods I used to stay off of most of the medications prescribed by my doctor

After recovering from cataract surgery, I decided to come up with a plan to lose weight and get back in shape. My goal was to get within 15 pounds of my high school weight and restart my life. As part of my plan to stay off of toxic medications, I only started on just two of the five drugs prescribed by my physician, with an ultimate goal to be on none. In addition, I went to a health food store and purchased a multivitamin and multimineral product to aid in the recovery process.

Next, I explored the web in search of a plan that would provide me with the best results in the shortest amount of time. I consulted with dietitians, friends, and relatives in the medical field. I read books and conducted research on the subjects. I left no stone unturned.

This plan had to include healthy solutions to weight loss and exercise while implementing measurable and attainable goals. We all know that as with most diet and exercise plans, people tend to start them very motivated for a few weeks then quit either because of weak or slow results. Therefore, this plan had to show results quickly while not further compromising my health. I was anal about monitoring every event. I checked my weight twice a day, my blood sugar three times a day and created a journal of what I ate, when and how much. These practices proved to be beneficial in keeping me focused and motivated in the long run.

Once again, I would like to mention I am not a physician, so please consult your healthcare provider before beginning a diet and exercise plan. What I have done is to essentially compile several remedies and exercises that when combined were very effective and allowed me to lose over 65 pounds in just six months. I saw my A1C, blood pressure, cholesterol and most importantly my weight drop rapidly.

Chapter *1*

Paradigm Shift

Mental toughness is the strength of mind that enables a person to encounter danger or bear pain or adversity with courage. Before anyone begins a diet and exercise program, I think they should examine their approach to dealing with adversity and search deep inside for the fortitude necessary to be successful. That won't happen until you change the mindset that got you in the predicament that you are in, to begin with.

I pledged a fraternity in college and one of the first lessons I learned was, "whatever can be mentally conceived can be physically achieved." Believe me, I had to reach for the inspiration that the phrase provided daily to complete the pledge process. The same can be said for my diet and exercise program. Given my poor diagnosis, I reached back to some of the life lessons that made me successful in the past. I knew if I didn't change my outlook on health and continued with the same old mindset, I was not going to achieve the desired results.

That brings me to a little story that I am going to share with you. While at work one afternoon I ran into a couple of colleagues that I hadn't seen me since my weight loss, and they ask me how I did it. These two ladies were clearly overweight and were open to discussing their weight issues. So, I essentially gave them an abbreviated version of my diet plan verbally, of course. One lady was extremely receptive and wanted me to write down my program, share more with her and help to monitor her progress. I agreed. The other lady literally found fault with almost everything I suggested. She was definitely indoctrinated to a failed belief system.

All I heard was one negative comment after the next. She made comments like "I don't know about giving up my red velvet cake." I took a good look at her and said to myself, "you will be fat for the rest of your life" simply because of your negative thought processes. In a similar example, a friend who also asked for help responded to my advice by assuring me she could not run for even 20 seconds to get the weight off. I ultimately advised her to walk if she couldn't run. The point here is to do something, anything. Stop, making excuses and get started. I shook my head but then quickly realized that I had that same mindset until I almost passed out walking up that infamous hill. It wasn't too long ago that my son's coach who saw me working out during practice, told me to trot or run instead of walking around the track. And you already know the answer, right? I told him I couldn't do it, it was too much. So, with all that in mind, I decided that I would encourage my friends rather than give up on them. Let's face it; most of us are wired like the ladies who responded negatively, myself included, and it may take a catastrophic event for us to realize that a change needs to take place. Essentially that is what happened to me, so I am not even remotely judgmental here.

The net of it is, no one is going to begin a transformation process until their mind is in the right place.

In 1980, Bob Marley released the popular reggae tune, "Redemption Song." He adapted this quote from a 1937 Marcus Garvey speech:

"Emancipate yourselves from mental slavery, none but ourselves can free our minds..."

That same thought process is very appropriate here. We are enslaved by our conventional approach to pharmaceuticals, food, and our way of thinking. And until we free our minds and toughen up a bit, we are just going to continue down the rabbit hole to disease and poor health. Thus, the first step after identifying that you actually have a weight problem is to alter the usual way of thinking and adopt a new approach that will bring about change. That my friend is what is known as a paradigm shift.

Exercise Your Mind

Before you exercise your body or exercise your arm by lifting the fork up to your mouth you should first exercise your mind. Many activities can help you change your perspective on weight loss and set you up for sustained success. Below I have named a few that should give you a quick start and help you along your journey.

1) Love on yourself: There is only one you and you are the captain of your ship. Show yourself some love. Smile and be positive. Find the best attributes that you possess and dwell on them.

2) Pump the breaks: In problem-solving, the first step is to acknowledge the problem. The same could be said about a paradigm shift. Stop, take a deep breath and admit that you have a health/weight problem, relax and think about your current mindset and then quickly discard.

3) Make it your own: Remember you are in control, only you hold the key to your success. When setting goals make them attainable and manageable. Make them your own.

4) Think on a higher level: Set fun goals that will ultimately give you your desired results without always focusing on weight loss. A good example would be to go out dancing or go hiking.

5) Don't be a secret agent: Whoever said you have to go it alone. Socialize weight loss and team up. Find an accountability partner. You may have gained weight all by yourself, but you don't have to lose it alone.

6) Think outside the square: Be unconventional, be a visionary. Have you ever heard of the definition of insanity? Just keep on doing what you have always done, and I guarantee you the results will be the same.

7) Nike Mentality: When all else fails "Just Do It." Don't wait for the New Year or some other event to take place. Stop making excuses and get started right now.

If you haven't noticed by now, just about all of the above steps involves exercising your mind. Your mindset is one of the, if the most critical assets in your weight loss arsenal, yet probably the most overlooked. Changing the way you think is an arduous yet necessary task to accomplish. I have confidence in you, exercise your mind, follow the rest of the program and reap the rewards.

Chapter 2

Cleansing

Now that your mind is in the right place, before moving on with a diet and exercise regimen you should conduct a whole-body cleanse. You didn't gain weight overnight, it took several years. The key thought here is how one could possibly lose weight if they don't remove the excess toxins that have built up over the years causing the body to slow down and contribute to bad health and weight gain.

When you begin a cleansing or detox program consider what got the toxins in your body in the first place. It's the environment which we have the least amount of control. It's what we eat and drink daily. In other words, it's what we put in our bodies either voluntary or involuntary over time.

Start off by first eliminating or cutting back on your toxin intake. Highly processed foods such as, sausages and hot dogs go through a manufacturing process which is filled with chemicals and toxins. Limit or eliminate all together alcohol. Quit smoking, monitor your coffee intake and of course stay away from energy drinks. Also, take in to account the harsh household chemicals, soaps, and shampoos you use daily. I'm not suggesting going through your kitchen and bathroom and discarding all your products in one fell swoop, but over time you can definitely seek more natural alternatives.

Here are 8 indicators that you may have excess toxins in the body:

(1) Weight gain

Have you gained weight over the years since high school? Have you tried diets before with poor results? You work out and work out even harder and never lose a pound. Good results may be hard to come by because of the toxins in your food

(2) Digestive Issues

If you are constantly bloated or suffer from constipation, check with your doctor, but it could be something as simple as a toxin in your gut. When you are constipated, it's very difficult for the body to remove all the stored toxins in your system.

(3) Headaches

So, you have been to the doctor for headaches, and she tells you there is nothing wrong. But you know all too well how you feel. You are always taking over the counter pain relievers, yet you can't seem to shake that headache. It could be because of the buildup of toxins in your body.

(4) Constant Fatigue

You get plenty of rest; you even go to the gym periodically, and you find it hard to finish a physical task without resting. It could be that your body is expending too much energy trying to get rid of the toxins you have put in it. So, what do you do next? You turn to energy drinks and put even more unwanted chemicals into your body. Not a good idea!

(5) Muscle Aches and Pains

If you work out or engage in strenuous activities, then there is the likelihood that you may have a few aches and pains. What if you don't work out yet your muscles ache, you believe it's just a natural part of aging right? It very well could be. It also could be toxins that are causing your body to ache.

(6) Puffy Eyes

Sure, puffy eyes could be because of a lack of sleep. My solution would be to try your best to get 6-8 hours' worth of sleep every night. Or maybe you could even take power naps during the day. If you are, however, getting enough rest and your eyes are still puffy. It's probably due to what you are eating.

(7) Halitosis (Bad breath) and Body Odor

You brush your teeth twice day floss and use mouth wash; you take frequent showers, and your co-workers give you an all in one body wash & shampoo along with a ten pack of breath mints for your birthday. That's probably a good indication that you have BO and halitosis. Guess what? You already know the answer. TOXINS!

(8) Skin Problems

The skin is the largest organ in the body, and when it's trying to tell us something, we should listen. Have you noticed adult acne or other skin rashes? Again, check with your dermatologist first, but disorders of the skin that manifest themselves on the surface of the body could be due to something going on internally. Like toxins.

My Cleansing Preferences

There are several different types of body cleanse programs available from capsules to shakes to teas. You name it, it's out there. Simply choose one or several and stick with it. My personal preference is the Detox, and Flush Whole Body Cleanse by "Natural Herbs." This product may aid with cleansing the liver, kidneys, colon, blood, pancreas, prostate, stomach and joints. It is also known to help with parasites and inflammation in the body. I took this shake once a day for 21 days, and it melted away pounds of sludge. Additionally, I took supplements such as milk thistle and dandelion root to also aid in the cleansing process.

Once again starting a diet and exercise program without eliminating harmful toxins in the body is like skydiving without a parachute. You wouldn't do that, would you? Alright Then! Apply that same thought process here. Cleanse then diet and reap the benefits.

Chapter 3

Home Remedies

I want you to think about your grandparents for a second. If your grandparents are like mine, then you heard a multitude of stories about how we have it easy today as they had to walk miles to school, didn't have central air or even a color TV. What you also heard were stories about how they came up with solutions to health problems by using home remedies. If I got sick while visiting my grandmother, she was famous for going in the back yard and picking something growing on a vine, boiling it and telling me to drink it. It certainly didn't kill me. It actually made me feel better.

I wish I would have bottled and marketed some of her home remedies. If I had, I would be sitting on a beach somewhere in the Caribbean right now. What is remarkable, however, is some health food companies are now beginning to recognize the health benefits of home remedies and are mass producing some of the same things that grandma used to give me. Aloe Vera comes to mind. It grew in our back yard, and we used it for cuts, bruises, and burns. Now it's a multimillion- dollar entity. As with any unconventional method of healing, critics are going to tell you there are not enough studies to substantiate our claims. I'm living proof that they actually work.

Let's begin by taking a look at a few solutions that are known to promote weight loss, cleanse the body and help to eradicate some of the unwanted diseases associated with obesity. We can do this by looking at products that you are probably already familiar with:

• **Aloe Vera**

Speaking of Aloe Vera, it certainly tops my list. It helps the body to remove toxins and can stimulate your metabolism. Get two leaves, remove the pulp, add to your favorite non-caloric beverage and blend for a few minutes. Drink daily

- **Green Tea**

Studies suggest that green tea can boost metabolism and promote weight loss. Drink a cup once or twice daily or drink it chilled instead of traditional iced tea.

- **Bitter Melon Fruit**

Some studies show that bitter melon fruit, tea or extract reduces blood sugar levels and improves glucose tolerance. Try drinking the tea after meals high in carbohydrates.

- **Lemon Juice**

Lemon Juice is known to remove toxins from the body and help promote proper digestion. It also has fat burning capabilities. Mix with honey and take a couple of teaspoons daily.

- **Apple Cider Vinegar**

Try adding organic apple cider vinegar to your daily regiment as well. 1-2 tablespoon a day of ACV in 8 ounces of water before meals has been known to aid in weight loss and stimulate digestion.

- **Juicing**

Consider drinking plenty of water and juicing green drinks as much as possible. You can juice kale, spinach or any green vegetable, just add a little fruit and fiber (nuts, flaxseed, etc.) and Bob's your uncle.

Flat Belly Diet

This next cleansing program was recommended to me a by an herbalist. In the past, no matter how much I exercised or dieted I was unable to shed the good old "beer belly." This go around. I went into a health food store and asked the herbalist for a product that would help me lose the "spare tire." She told me she would love to sell me a product, but there was no need to and that I probably had the solution and ingredients I needed to solve my problem already at home. She recommended that I try a cleansing program called the "Flat Belly Diet." Let me emphasize that I take no credit for the development of this diet I merely looked it up online, tried it and I can attest to it....it actually works.

Here It Is:

- 2 liters water
- 1 teaspoon freshly grated ginger.
- 1 medium cucumber peeled and thinly sliced.
- 1 medium lemon thinly sliced.
- 12 small peppermint leaves.
- Combine all ingredients in a large pitcher and let flavors blend overnight.
- Drink the entire pitcher by the end of each day
- Drink three days straight

I'm not sure how or why it works, but it does cleanse the body and reduce belly bloat. When you look at the ingredient individually, they start to paint a picture of health. The moral of the story is; remember to cleanse and Detox your body and give yourself a fighting chance to succeed before beginning a diet and exercise program.

Heart Blockage or Cholesterol Lowering Tonic

How I came about this home remedy is rather interesting. I was on the phone with a friend, and my doctor's office called. I put my buddy on hold and took the call. Of course, it was terrible news. My cholesterol numbers came back elevated, and it was suggested that I start immediately on a statin. You already know I didn't do that. I took my call off of hold and continued talking to my buddy. He could sense that something was wrong, so I decided to share my condition with him. He quickly said not to worry; he would send me a link to a cholesterol-lowering remedy that I could try. Again, I take no credit for how this remedy came about. I can, however, tell you that it worked, and I have the labs to prove it. Some people refer to it as the "miracle cure." I don't know about that, but it does works.

Be prepared to open the windows and turn on the fans in your home as you will experience a strong and pungent odor while preparing this tonic. Grab the clothespin for your nose and let's go!

Ingredients:

- Ginger Juice – 1 cup
- Garlic Juice – 1 cup
- Lemon Juice – 1 cup
- Apple Cider Vinegar – 1 cup
- Honey – 3 cups

How to prepare:

1. Take ginger juice, garlic juice, lemon juice and vinegar in a saucepan and cook on medium heat for 30 minutes. Mix frequently.
2. Cool it completely.
3. Add in 3 cups of honey and mix well (Add the Honey only after cooling the mixture).
4. Pour this into a clean glass bottle and store in a refrigerator (This tonic can be stored for up to two months).

Note: I found the best way to get a cup of garlic juice was to use a food processor. A blender will produce more of a puree and will add an additional step to your preparation. If you must use a blender, then take the puree and strain through a cheesecloth. Please only use organic raw ACV.

How to use:

Take 1 tablespoon of this medicine on an empty stomach every morning. You can also take an additional tablespoon at night before bedtime.

Last but not least Go organic. There are several advantages to using organic products.

- Organic fruits and vegetables are grown with fewer pesticides
- Organic food doesn't contain preservatives. Therefore they are fresher
- Organic meat, dairy, and eggs don't contain hormones, antibiotics and are GMO-free.

Whether you decide to go organic or not always remember to use a fruit and vegetable wash. These products remove wax, pesticides, and chemicals from your food.

Chapter 4

Food and Diet

We now live in a microwave, fast food and smartphone era where everything including the way we eat can be consumed almost instantaneously. Heck, we can now even use an app on our smartphones to have food delivered to us just about anywhere we like. Progress is a beautiful thing but not at the expense of our health. Our fast-paced lifestyle has undoubtedly led to a shift in our eating patterns. It has pretty much caused us to eat processed foods high in refined sugars, saturated fats, and sodium. Moreover, we are not eating enough fruit, vegetables, and fiber to maintain a healthy diet. This lifestyle change has put us on a crash course with you guessed it, diabetes, hypertension, hyperlipidemia, and even cancer.

Let's begin by addressing three very unhealthy substances that we should try and avoid as much as possible if not eliminate altogether. This is obviously not an extensive list, however; they are the usual suspects in what we consume in this fast-paced world we live in.

• Sugars

Sugar in excess is known to promote obesity. We as a society definitely overindulge in our sugar consumption. Sugar is in our morning cereals, fruit drinks, sodas, adult beverages, cookies, cakes and condiments such as ketchup Just to name a few.

• Salt/Sodium

Salt is the silent killer and is linked to hypertension and heart disease. Excess salt is found in snack foods, sauces, processed meats, and most take-out foods.

• **Fats**

Intake of saturated fats can promote weight gain, high cholesterol and can lead to other diseases associated with metabolic syndrome. High concentrations of fat are usually associated with animal products such as red meats, processed meats, and some oils.

To eat healthily, we must choose an eating pattern that encompasses the five essential food groups which are dairy, fruits, grains, proteins, and vegetables. If you can find a way, incorporate these foods into your daily diet, and you will be well on your way to eating healthy.

My Diet Plan

At first, I thought about going vegan and trust me, I know the health benefits of doing so. I am going to eventually get there, but if you are like me, it just might take a few months. My diet plans on the other hand, while not vegan did eliminate several foods that I absolutely love to eat. My plan is relatively simple. I did nothing outrageous nor did I implement any dietary changes that were unsustainable. I used a common-sense approach to lose weight from a food perspective.

Terrified by the poor long-term prognosis of diabetes and hypertension, I knew immediately that I had to cut the carbs, sugar and table salt out of my diet. Interestingly enough l found it almost impossible to eat anything that didn't contain carbs. Remember Low- carbs does not mean no-carbs. There are plenty of carbs in vegetables by the way. With that in mind, I literally cut out all rice, pasta, bread, dairy, snack foods (cakes, cookies, chips, etc.), vegetable oils and most of all processed and red meats from my meals.

Additionally, I eliminated alcohol, all sodas, and fruit drinks and substituted them with no calorie seltzers. I also refrained from eating any condiments or sauces (fish oil, teriyaki, etc.)

You might be wondering, *so what the heck did he eat.* Ok, you twisted my arm, I will tell you. I ate fish high in omega-3s like salmon, codfish, mackerel baked or broiled of course. I did eat hard boiled eggs as well.

I used olive oil, sesame seed oil, avocado oil, and sea salt in my foods. I used riced cauliflower (found in the freezer section of your local supermarket). I ate leafy green vegetables such as brussels sprouts, broccoli, spinach, and kale. To add a little starch to my balanced meal, I added small portions of corn and/or sweet potatoes. I did eat some fruit, mostly green apples, and blueberries but only for breakfast or a snack and before 12 noon. Since fruit, while a healthy choice, contains sugars I limited my consumption to before noon. I also incorporated nuts and legumes into my diet plan. I stuck to this regiment for the first three months with unbelievable results.

As I noticed the weight dropping off, I decided to have a life again, and I began to add back in a few things. I added back some dairy and soy or almond milk; I added brown rice, multigrain pasta and sprouted bread, all in moderation of course. I also added back in some red wines as well. So, you see not bad at all but, remember I was a fanatic for the first 90 days. I didn't waver at all from my diet plan. Even though I added back in a few comfort foods, I still limited my consumption of them for the second 90-day period.

We touched on what kinds of foods that helped me lose weight, now allow me to share with you how. In real estate, they say buying and selling successfully is dependent upon location, location, and location. As far as dieting is concerned, it's all about portion control. It doesn't matter what you eat or how often, if you overindulge when you do.

I purchased a plate from the dollar store that was divided into three, and I used it to section off my food and control my portion size. You know that little plate you used to put your kids' meals on?

Yeah, that one. I put meat in one section, vegetables in the other and starch in the third (very little starch if any). If it couldn't fit in the plate, I didn't eat it.

In addition, I tried to limit my carbs to less than 35 grams per meal. Yes, I counted carbs. If you read labels which I did, they will tell you how many carbs each serving contains.

Now, you may be wondering if I ate out at all while dieting. Absolutely yes! Dieting is not a death sentence. If you are not having some type of fun during the process, then you probably will quit before you see the results. So, eat out if you wish. What I did though, was to stick to my meal plan of mostly fish and vegetables. At restaurants, I would immediately ask for a to-go box when my meal arrived and saved half for another day. That also saved money. Just remember to practice self-control and do all things in moderation.

Chapter 5

Stress Relief

Stress can be very damaging to anyone. Whether its stress from work, stress from marriage or stress for financial reasons; it can hurt the body. When a person is stressed, hormones are released that prepare the body to fight or flee. The release of these hormones ultimately impacts the insulin in the blood and can elevate glucose levels among other things... critical if you are diabetic. According to the Mayo Clinic, "It may be those other behaviors linked to stress — such as overeating, drinking alcohol and poor sleeping habits — that can cause high blood pressure. However, short-term stress-related spikes in your blood pressure added up over time may put you at risk of developing long-term high blood pressure."

Overeating, unhealthy eating habits and/or drinking alcohol in excess can naturally lead to weight gain or make it very difficult to lose the pounds you have already acquired. Just think when you are stressed out, do you reach for celery or carrots? I don't think so. The body craves salty and sweet foods like chips, cake or ice cream. When was the last time you saw a friend who was stress from a break –up eating a healthy snack? With all this in mind, it is imperative that we find a way to reduce the stress in our lives or we can pretty much count out losing weight and getting healthy. There seems to be a trend developing here. There are so many factors that may have contributed to your weight loss difficulties of the past, but we have it covered here.

There are many ways to reduce or elevate stress. I have listed 10 examples:

1. Meditate or take Yoga Lessons

I like to call meditation adult timeout. It allows an individual to find a quiet space and take charge of their own emotions. This time belongs to you so own it and reap the spiritual and health benefits it has to offer.

2. Exercise

Not only will exercise aid in the weight loss process but, it's a fact that exercise release hormones in your body called endorphins, which are natural pain and stress fighters. These hormones are known to trigger a positive feeling in the body.

3. Bump some tunes

You have heard the saying that "music tames the savage beast." Well, it's actually true, very true. There are numerous studies out there that prove music reduces the levels of the stress hormone cortisol.

4. Talk about it

Sometimes it actually an excellent idea to contact a friend, vent and get your problem off of your chest. Find a peer group or a spiritual advisor and talk about your situation. In other words, just release!

5. Find a hobby

Again, own this process. You are always trying to please your loved ones, your boss and others. Find something YOU like to do and start a new hobby. I don't know, collect trains or baby dolls, but do something for you.

6. Adopt a pet

Pet therapy is becoming very popular. Studies show that playing with or petting an animal can increase the levels the hormone oxytocin which plays a role in decreasing the production of cortisol. There goes that cortisol (stress) hormone again.

7. Volunteer-read to children or the elderly

Get out of the house and volunteer. There are plenty of skilled nursing facilities and elementary schools that would love for you to come out and read to their residents and students. Being of service to others can be a stress reducer in and of itself.

8. Read a book

You have just read to someone else now try reading a book for yourself. Find a topic you like, for example, cooking or reading a spy novel. You decide but do something. Reading can reduce stress by allowing you to relax and get away for a few minutes.

9. Drink herbal teas

Peppermint and Chamomile teas are known for their stress reducing and calming effects. They work to relax the muscles and fight off anxiety. Try a cup instead of pulling your hair out.

10. Laugh out loud

Laugh out loud...I wouldn't do this in public by the way. You just might get a few strange stares if you do. Have you ever heard the saying, "laugh and the world laughs with you"? Try it, learn to laugh at your own situations and watch, others will laugh with you instead of at you.

My Stress Relievers

You can try most if not all of the above stress relievers with minimal effort and yet yield huge rewards. While I participated in most I, however, found different forms of meditation to be very easy to implement, cost-effective and absolutely rewarding. You don't have to be an expert, a guru or even take expensive yoga classes to begin a meditation program on your own and at home. Now, I know this may seem kind of corny to most guys, I know, I know but, just try it no one has to know, trust me, a little quiet time can go a long way, and she will like you better when you lose the weight. While there may be thousands of ways to meditate, I tried a few, and they worked well.

The Atmosphere

I started out by first finding a quiet place in my home, which I know can be almost impossible to do at times. Nevertheless, I made it happen. The goal here is to find a place where you would be uninterrupted for about 30 minutes. People use various techniques; I say employ the KISS method, "keep it simple stupid." Sit on the floor, a bed, in a chair or wherever just have your back upright and be comfortable.

Aromatherapy

Again, not a guru here but several fragrances help relax the body and put the mind at ease. I will name a few essential oils here. Again, guys bear with me no one is going to pull your man card if you meditate.

- Frankincense: is believed to help you connect with your inner spirit.
- Cedarwood: allows you to focus inward
- Sandalwood: helps you to heal emotionally and spiritually
- Rose: is known to open your heart and help promote self-love

Now, how you chose to administer the scents is entirely up to you, some people use candles and others actually burn incense, I used a diffuser and tried a different oil until I found the one that worked best for me.

Close your eyes and focus

There are several meditation methods. I chose the concentration method where I concentrated on one thought for the duration of my session. It may be a little challenging to start out. As with most new things, give it a chance, try 5 minutes then work your way up to a half hour. Breathe in and breathe out slowly. Don't try to control your breathing, just allow it to occur naturally.

Music and Meditation

You can also use music to employ the concentration method. Choose your genres and get started. I particularly like reggae music. The trick here is to concentrate or focus on a single aspect of the music. I love the beat. I canceled everything out and concentrated on the drums and before you know it 30 minutes were up and I was relaxed. That brings me to my next point; time your sessions.

Cooking can be a form of Meditation

If all else fails, try to combine a few of the methods. I like to cook. Cooking relaxes me, especially when once again I can tune everyone and everything out. Try putting on a pair of headphones and commence to prepare a healthy meal. Cooking with herbs like rosemary can help with the relaxation process as well.

Find which stress reliever works best for you. The point is to choose one or combine several. Take some time out for yourself, and you will begin to reap the benefits of a stress-free life.

Chapter 6

Fasting

First of all, what is fasting?

"Fasting is a willing abstinence or reduction from some or all food, drink or both, for a period of time."- Wikipedia.

Fasting can be done for a religious reason or in our case to promote weight loss. Just think we all already practice this ancient ritual but seemed to have forgotten or were never taught the health benefits. Where do you think the word breakfast comes from, you guessed it from fasting? Your morning meal is merely a form of breaking your fast from your meal consumed the night before, hence the term *Break-fast* = Breakfast.

Fasting Myths

Let's be clear starving yourself is the last thing I would recommend, however, fasting in moderation can provide numerous health benefits. Before we jump into some of these benefits, let's first dispel a few myths associated with fasting:

- Fasting puts the body in starvation mode
- Skipping meals will slow down your metabolism
- Fasting causes muscle loss
- Fasting causes the brain to malfunction

First of all, we already fast by not eating for 8 hours or more between dinner and breakfast. So, I don't know if there is even a need to go further but, I will. Fasting is simply a decision of what time of the day to eat or how often to eat in a given timeframe. Starvation, on the other hand, is a deficiency in caloric intake over a period of time. The operative word in all of this is "time."

Next, let's explore the effects of skipping meals on our metabolism. There is a paradigm shift that needs to be employed here. Conventional wisdom tells us that we need to have breakfast first thing in the morning, lunch around noon and dinner in the evenings to maintain healthy eating habits. There is absolutely no proof that changing your eating style will negatively impact your metabolism. Fasting In fact actually increases several fat burning hormones that help regulate growth and metabolism.

Can fasting cause muscle loss, probably if you starve yourself for an extended period? I am obviously not suggesting starvation here just fasting. Changing your meal frequency or changing the time that you eat won't hurt your muscles. The relationship between proteins and muscle is quite interesting. Amino acids found in food are the building blocks of protein. It is true, however; that amino acids found in muscle can be converted into energy if food is depleted. There is no benefit to your body by getting more protein than it can use. Your body takes the protein it needs and burns off excess energy, excretes it or stores the extra calories as fat.

Again, I believe people are more than likely using the words fasting and starvation interchangeably especially as it relates to the brain. There is a lot of information that suggests that fasting can negatively impact the brain because it lacks fuel stores and therefore requires a continuous supply of glucose to function properly. Scientifically there may be some truth to that statement if there are prolonged periods of fasting. Consider the opposite. When we consume large meals during Thanksgiving or other holidays, don't we tend to get sleepy and become lethargic? The most we can do is yell at our TV's and cheer for our favorite football team, right? Are our brains functioning at full capacity in that scenario? I don't think so. But when we are hungry, do we just shut down give up and pass out or are our brains functioning on all cylinders trying to figure out ways to find food? Hmm! Just scorer the web and you will find numerous articles on how the brain actually rejuvenates and cleanses itself after brief periods of fasting.

Benefits of Intermittent Fasting

Intermittent fasting, first of all, is abstaining or reducing food or drink intake periodically. It is not a diet but merely a change in our pattern of eating. There are many health benefits associated with intermittent fasting including weight loss, lower blood pressure, and reduced cholesterol. It's also been known to reduce fat and create lean muscle.

The good news is that when engaging in intermittent fasting, there is no need to change what we eat or how many calories we intake on a daily basis. Again, the key here is to change when we eat. This concept should allow us to get started on a fasting program rather easily and stay on it until our results are achieved. The most challenging task is to change our mindset from the conventional way of consuming our meals. To put it in perspective, intermittent fasting is entirely in your control. You can start and stop as you wish. It is not necessary to be regimented when implementing a fasting program. If your buddy comes into town and wants to get some hot wings and beer, are you going to say sorry I'm fasting right now? I know I'm probably going to indulge. You see I have complete control over when, where and how I fast. What I would do in that scenario is to simply change my fasting period.

Types of Intermittent Fasting

There are many types of intermittent fasting methods. Some are more difficult to implement than others; while some may not work well with the old 9-5 or the kids' schedules. Chose the one that best fits your lifestyle and give it a try.

• The 16/8 Method

Basically, fast for 16 hours each day. This is not that different from what we already do now. Now we probably eat dinner around 7pm and fast until breakfast around 7am or thereabouts. This method can easily be achieved by eating our last meal for the evening at 7pm and not eating again until 11am the next day.

This method is also known as the Leangains protocol made popular by Martin Berkhan. Feel free to drink coffee, water or non-caloric flavored waters to help with the hunger pangs.

- **The 5/2 Method**

This method also known as the fast diet was made famous by Dr. Michael Mosley and can be implemented rather quickly. Eat normally for 5 days of the week and restrict calories to 500-600 the other 2 days of the week.

- **The Warrior Diet**

This method involves eating very little during the day, only consuming small amounts of raw fruits and vegetables; then during the evening eating a huge meal. This method was developed by fitness expert Ori Hofmekler.

- **Eat Stop Eat**

This next method is essentially a 24-hour fasting program. Fast for 24 hours once or twice a week. During this period consume no food. Again, water and other non-caloric beverages can be consumed.

So, for example, if you eat dinners at 6pm on the first night, then don't eat again until dinner at 6pm the next evening. You can also choose to fast from lunch to lunch or breakfast to breakfast. This method was made popular by Brad Pilon.

- **Alternate Day Diet**

This diet was popularized by Dr. James Johnson and is very easy to implement. This is how it works: Eat minimal one day, keeping your caloric intake between 400 and 500. And then eat normally the next.

- **Randomized Fasting**

Randomized fasting is a method that most working people or people with active kids already practice and don't even know it. Just merely skip a meal every now and then or if you miss a meal don't try to make it up. Most people who practice this method do so by skipping breakfast. Don't buy into the myth that breakfast is the most important meal of the day. If you have stopped growing, there is no need for breakfast.

My Fasting Method

After reviewing the various methods listed above, I decided to implement the "Eat Stop Eat" program. At first, it was tough to wrap my arms around not eating for 24 hours. Once I got started, however, it became second nature.

I would start off on a Saturday and eat three meals for the day, consuming my last meal around 6pm. The next day I would not eat until Sunday dinner at 6pm. On Monday I would eat three meals again ending at 6pm and fast on Tuesday, and so on and so one for a total of 3 fasting days during the week.

I found this plan to be very rewarding and quite refreshing. I had a lot more energy and would drop five pounds every time I applied this method. The keys to success were to stay busy during the fasting period, exercise, stay in my daily routine and actually sleep through as much of it as possible. Also, I would drink plenty of carbonated water to stave off hunger. One of the biggest takeaways of the "Eat Stop Eat" program is to remember NOT to overindulge when you do eat. Eat a regular meal as if you didn't fast for 24 hours.

Intermittent fasting actually works if we can get beyond the anxiety of actually trying it. Your friends and colleagues are going to try to discourage you. So-called experts are going to tell you everything that could possibly go wrong. Just keep in mind that you are not starving yourself, you are just changing the frequency or pattern of eating.

Chapter 7

Exercise and Fitness Program

Allow me to start off by sharing with you an example of what I experienced over the years regarding exercise and tell me if it sounds familiar. If you are anything like me, and the folks I associate with, you exercise seasonally. You start a workout program, do it for a while, stop it and start all over again and then wonder why you haven't lost any weight. During the week I would walk around the track with several parents while we waited for our kids to finish with football practice. Then on Saturday I would eat pizza and drink beers & margaritas after the games. You know what I am going to say next right? ....and wondered why I didn't lose any weight. The point here is to exercise (no pun intended) some common sense. Why shed a few pounds during the week and pile back on a bunch of empty calories during the weekend. Be disciplined my friend, be disciplined.

Now on a more positive note, we can fix our weight gain issues and embark on a journey to good health and fitness. Our exercise and workout routine is the last yet, one of the most essential steps in the weight loss process. As with diets, I can tell you from a personal standpoint that maintaining a sound exercise program can be a daunting task. But it really shouldn't be at all. Once again, the hardest part is making the mental adjustment to actually get off the couch and shed your sedentary lifestyle. Shed the mindset, and you will drop the pounds. It's that simple. I'm living proof.

I'm sure you have seen a ton of infomercials on TV describing how their workout program can help you lose weight just in time for your high school reunion. I bet you have also seen the commercials with actors who are already in shape with rock hard abs, pushing expensive exercise equipment. You may have even purchased a program or fitness machine yourself. If you have, tell the truth it's probably under your bed gathering dust, right? Or you used it to no avail.

Now, don't get me wrong I'm not trying to dissuade you from purchasing something that can assist you with your weight loss goals. If a program or exercise machine works for you, I say go for it. Honestly, though, it is entirely unnecessary to spend a lot of money or join an expensive gym. Beginning an exercise and fitness program can be as easy or as difficult as you want it to be. My suggestion is to keep it simple and save money.

There are a plethora of programs at your disposal. I can't even begin to name all of them. The net of it is to do something, anything! And remember to cleanse first and then run the next 5 steps of our weight loss program concurrently.

I am now going to touch on four popular programs and then share with you my personal approach to exercise.

CrossFit

CrossFit is an exercise program created by Greg Glassman. It is essentially a high-intensity program that provides a full body workout by combining movements in gymnastics, weightlifting, running, rowing and more. Not to worry, it can be designed to suit anyone from the elite athlete to beginner. There are also home-based methods available as well.

HIIT or High-Intensity Interval Training

HIIT is known to rapidly burn calories in a short period. It can be performed using a treadmill, running on a track or just running in place in your living room. You can jump rope, do jumping jacks or just about anything. You decide what works best for you. The idea is to go full throttle for a short period followed by a short period of rest.

Dance Routines

Zumba comes to mind when I think of a dance fitness program. It was created by Columbian dancer Alberto Perez. There are similar dance programs available, and they can be found anywhere from your cable TV network to online videos. It is a fun way to burn calories without even realizing it by dancing and listening to great music.

Running Program

An effective running program starts off slow. You didn't just wake up overweight one day. It occurred over time. Apply that same logic to your running program. Run for a few minutes then stop or run then trot then walk. Just drink plenty of water, briefly rest in between runs and increase your time or distance gradually.

My Actual Workout Routine

I promised you I would share my actual work out plan so here it goes:

I began by walking in my subdivision. Fortunately, I live in a big complex with lots of hills. I walked 3-5 times a week from my house to the beginning of the complex and back for about three weeks. Once I mastered walking the neighborhood, I decided that I needed something with a little more intensity, so I downloaded an app on my phone called "Couch to 5K" by Zenlabs Fitness. To be honest, I have no intentions of ever running a 5K. My goal was to uses a program that was intense, structured, timed, repetitive and measurable. And that app provided me with all the tools I needed to get off the couch and shed the pounds.

Primarily, the program was a form of HIIT. I would warm up; run or trot briefly, followed by a brief period of walking, repeated the steps and then cooled down. I followed the program and repeated the routine for several weeks until I was in shape. I will say it's not necessary to follow the program completely. Repeat weeks if need be or even walk rapidly if you are not ready to run. Again, take advantage of the tools it has to offer and stick to a plan, your plan.

The app is designed to be used three times a week; then it increases in intensity from week one to week nine. That was all good but, after a few weeks of losing weight, I need to pick up the pace and add another routine. I decided to do a "Burpee" workout with shadow boxing, followed by a rest period the other two days of the week. Let me explain:

Burpee with Push-Up & Shadow Boxing Intervals

If that sounds pretty intense and difficult, you guessed it, you are right it is! But there goes that mindset thing again. If it can be mentally conceived, then it can be psychically done.

Burpee with a pushup:

1. Begin in a squat position with hands on the floor in front of you.
2. Kick your feet back, while simultaneously lowering yourself into the bottom portion of a pushup.
3. Immediately return your feet to the squat position, while simultaneously pushing "up" with your arms. You will perform a pushup as you return your feet to the squat position.
4. Leap up as high as possible from the squat position.
5. Repeat, moving as fast as possible.

- Burpees x 30 seconds
- Shadowbox x 30 seconds
- Continue the entire process for 2 minutes
- Rest for 3-5 minutes

The object here is not to use the shadow boxing as a rest period but to use it as an enhancement to the Burpee interval.

I actually kept the whole process going for six months as I watched the pounds fall right off. I would occasionally change the days I performed the routines, but nevertheless, I got it in.

Chapter 8

Weight Management Program

Okay, you have followed a weight loss program, and it worked. You are in shape, and all your labs came back normal. You are feeling pretty good about yourself right now. But wait, not so fast. I don't mean to discourage you, but more than likely you are just going to revert back to your old habits and gain the weight back in no time. Keeping excess weight off can be a constant battle, very similar to what alcoholic and drug abusers go through.

You know by now the importance of mental toughness and how developing the right mindset can go a long way in helping you lose and keep off unwanted pounds. I bet you didn't know that there is a lot more to weight management than meets the eye. Studies show that over 80% of dieters will regain weight within a year or two of losing it. Guess what? It may not entirely be their fault; the body fights back and releases hormones that actually encourage them to gain the weight right back.

So what is the solution then? Let's employ some logic. Bad habits and a sedentary lifestyle created the problem. A paradigm shift, mental toughness, a healthy lifestyle, and exercise allowed you to lose weight, right? There is good news after all. There are also studies that prove that individual who remain focused and follow a maintenance program can actually keep the weight off for a lifetime. Here are a few ideas that may help:

- Monitor your weight periodically
- Recognize shift in your eating patterns
- Be aware of how your clothes fit

- Cleanse periodically
- Implement a fasting program when needed
- Exercise more than you eat

These simple tips can go a long way to beating the odds, staying in shape and looking good for the rest of your life.

My Maintenance Plan

My overall maintenance goal is to tone up by building lean muscle and getting rid of some of the loose skin that appeared after weight loss. By continuing a workout routine and staying focused I can rest assured that the excess weight won't return. With that in mind, I have implemented a rather simple plan; I exercise roughly five times a week. If I miss a day no worries, I rarely try to make it up. My routine combines cardio and resistance training which promotes continued fat loss, muscle tone and a strong core (great abs).

Cardio for me involves a brief warm-up followed by brisk walking, stadiums or very and I mean very short sprints. This routine almost guarantees that I will tone my core and lower body while increasing my heart rate. Every other day I focus on my upper body and once again my core or midsection via resistance training. Dumbbells and resistance bands are inexpensive methods that can apply an opposing force and build muscle. Additionally, I use my own bodyweight to produce results by doing push-ups, lunges, planks, and arm raises. Always remember stretch, warm up and cool down. Good Luck!

Conclusion

Look at Me Now!

It's funny how weight loss can improve just about every aspect of your life. The obvious improvement is your health but, there are several other intended or unintended benefits to weight loss. When I gained weight, the opposite sex stopped noticing me. Intimacy fell off a little. People, in general, were no longer taking me seriously. Now that I'm in shape and look 20 years younger I'm getting winks at the stoplight again. I'm kidding here a little, or maybe not. Being in shape and in good health has definitely impacted my life for the better. First of all, I no longer snore, and I sleep great. I have more confidence, I'm more assertive, and I have the energy to get off the couch and get things done. I have changed my wardrobe, well I had no choice my clothes no longer fit; I absolutely look better and feel better. What a difference six months can make.

Again, I would like to make it crystal clear that I'm not advocating firing your physician or never using prescribed medication again. What I am saying, however, is do the research on your prescribed medications. Ask your healthcare provider questions about your ailments and if it's safe to start an exercise and/or diet program. Ask about support groups in your area. Remember physicians are very busy and receive most of their education after med school from Pharma reps or from industry-funded clinical research and industry-funded seminars and continuing education programs.

Give your liver and kidneys a chance. Check with your doctor, put the remote control down, get off the couch and most of all stop smoking, drinking and eating excessively, (1) Change the way you think, (2) cleanse your body at least once every three months, (3) seek out nontoxic alternatives to medicine, (4) eat healthy, (5) eliminate stress in your life, (6) fast when you can, (7) exercise and (8) employ a maintenance program. Nothing in life is absolute except vodka, get the joke? But if you follow these 8 easy steps, you will be well on your way to a healthier productive and more rewarding life. Longevity is the key.

Appendix A

Sample Grocery List

Cut out all white processed foods!!!

- **Seafood/Meat:**
  - Lean grass-fed beef (only if you must), organic chicken breast
  - Fish--cod, salmon, trout, tuna, mackerel
  - Lean pork (only if you must), tofu

- **Bread/Grains/Pasta:**
  - Steel cut oatmeal, quinoa, brown rice (only if absolutely necessary), riced cauliflower, Ezekiel bread, ancient grain pasta, ancient grain cereals

- **Vegetables/Fruits:**
  - Leafy green vegetables- kale, spinach, swiss chard, arugula, mustard greens, collard greens, romaine lettuce
  - Broccoli, bell peppers, corn, carrots, zucchini, squash, onions, green onions/scallions, garlic, tomatoes, sweet potato, avocado
  - Berries, green apples, lemon, lime, grapes, watermelon, pineapple, ginger

- **Other:**
  - Bitter melon, low sodium organic peanut butter, cholesterol-friendly buttery spread

- **Diary/Non-Diary:**
  - Almond milk, mozzarella, parmesan, low-fat low sodium cheddar, nonfat Greek yogurt, organic brown eggs, soy milk

- **Nuts/Seeds:**
  - Almonds, walnuts, sunflower, pine nut, chia, flaxseed

- **Condiments/Oils & Vinegar:**
  - Olive oil-based mayo, olive oil, avocado oil, sesame oil
  - grapeseed oil, organic apple cider vinegar, pomegranate infused red wine vinegar

- **Snacks/Desserts:**
  - Toasty peanut butter crackers, celery, and peanut butter, carrot sticks, dried apricots, dates and figs

- **Beverages:**
  - Water, zero-calorie flavored seltzer water, low calorie no carb powered beverage mix

- **Teas:**
  - Bitter melon tea, moringa seed tea, soursop leaf tea, mint tea, chamomile tea

- **Sweeteners:**
  - Stevia, brown sugar (only if absolutely necessary)

- **Supplement List:**
  - Grapeseed extract, Vitamin E, Vitamin C, Milk thistle, Multi-vitamin/ multi-mineral, flaxseed, omega-3 fish oil, CoQ10, Vitamin D &magnesium, Tocotrienols

- **Herbs/Spices:**
  - Cinnamon, turmeric, thyme, oregano, black pepper, cayenne pepper, sea salt

- **Bean/ Legumes:**
  - Lentils, chickpeas, split peas, kidney beans, lima beans, black beans, black eye peas, pinto beans

Sample Meal Plan

❖ **Breakfast**

- Breakfast Smoothie
- A half cup of almond milk or a quarter cup of almonds
- A hand full of blueberries
- A quarter cup of Greek yogurt (only if you must)
- A tablespoon of ground flaxseed
- A hand full of kale
- Blend and enjoy.
- Hardboiled egg for protein

❖ **Mid- Morning Snack**

- Celery and peanut butter or green apple

❖ **Lunch**

- Lean chicken breast and a small salad

❖ **Dinner**

- A half cup of brown rice, baked salmon, six broccoli spears

❖ **After Dinner Snack**

- Carrot Sticks

Appendix B

Supplements

- **COQ10:** Protects the heart and blood vessels.
- **Flaxseed:** Reduces the risk of heart disease, cancer, stroke, and diabetes.
- **Grape Seed Extract:** May help improve circulation and cholesterol as well as other cardiovascular health.
- **Milk Thistle:** Provides heart benefits by lowering cholesterol levels. Helps diabetes in people who have type 2 diabetes and cirrhosis.
- **Multi-Vitamin/Multi-Mineral:** Used to treat or prevent vitamin deficiency due to poor diet and certain illnesses.
- **Omega-3 Fish Oil:** Helps lower blood pressure, reduce triglycerides, slow development of plaque in the arteries, reduce the chance of abnormal heart rhythm, reduce the likelihood of heart attack and stroke, and lessen the chance of sudden cardiac death in people with heart disease.
- **Tocotrienols:** Health benefits and may even affect how such illnesses as cardiovascular disease, diabetes, and certain kinds of cancer are treated in the future.

Appendix C

Sample Food & Activity Journal

Foods

Time of Day	Eat in or Take Out	Food Item	Number of Carbs	Calories

Activities

Time of Day	Activity	Duration

Daily Diary

SHED THE MINDSET SHED THE POUNDS

Sample Progress Tracker

Week 1	Date	Weight	Loss/Gain	Waist Circumf- erence	Blood Pressure	Blood Sugar
Week 2						
Week 3						

Appendix D

Glossary

- **Cardiovascular:** Relating to the heart and blood vessels
- **Carotid Artery:** Supply the head and neck with oxygenated blood
- **Cholesterol:** Is a waxy, fat-like substance that's found in all cells of the body.
- **Cortisol:** A steroid hormone that helps the body use sugar and fat for energy.
- **Hormones:** Chemical substances produced by body cells and released into the blood.
- **Hyperglycemia or High Blood Sugar:** Is a condition in which an excessive amount of glucose circulates in the blood plasma.
- **Hyperlipidemia:** An abnormally high concentration of fats or lipids in the blood.
- **Hypertension:** Abnormally high blood pressure.
- **Hypoglycemia or low blood:** Is when blood sugar decreases to below normal levels.
- **Ischemic Eye Disease:** Is a sudden loss of central vision, side vision or both due to a decreased or interrupted blood flow to the eye's optic nerve.
- **Metabolic Syndrome:** Is a cluster of conditions- Increased blood pressure, high blood sugar, excess body fat around the waist, and abnormal cholesterol or triglyceride levels- that occur together, increasing your risk of heart disease, stroke, and diabetes.
- **Mortality:** The state of being subject to death.
- **Obesity:** Condition of being grossly fat or overweight.
- **Oxytocin:** A powerful hormone that acts as a neurotransmitter in the brain.
- **Statins:** Class of drugs often prescribed by doctors to help lower cholesterol levels in the blood.

- **Triglycerides:** Type of fat in your body
- **Type 1 Diabetes:** Form of diabetes mellitus in which not enough insulin is produced. A chronic condition in which the pancreas produces little or no insulin.
- **Type 2 Diabetes:** Once known as adult-onset or noninsulin-dependent diabetes, is a chronic condition that affects the way your body metabolizes sugar (glucose), your body's essential source of fuel.